Kettlebell Workouts For Women:

Kettlebell Training and Exercise Book

By

Charles Maldonado

W0010666

978-1-68127-100-2

Table of Contents

Kettlebell Workouts For Women: Kettlebell Training
and Exercise Book

By Charles Maldonado

Introduction

Are you looking for excellent comprehensive workout, with limited equipment, that will get you results? A Kettlebell workout may be the right tool for you to get into shape and keep you in shape. Kettlebells look like a shot-put with a handle, but don't let appearances deceive you these weights deliver results.

Kettlebells are weights made of steel or cast-iron. Training with kettlebells can result in very impressive results and lead to improved balance, strength, power and aerobic abilities. With this one piece of equipment you can complete a vigorous total body work out.

Chapter 1. Benefits of Working Out with Kettlebells

Did you know that exercise builds bone mass? This is great for women. Women are more susceptible to Osteoporosis at the age of 50 and over. Exercise like working with kettlebells can help slow the aging process and strengthen your bones.

Kettlebells can be a great workout for people of all levels of fitness, genders and ages. For women, kettlebells can have a great number of benefits. Below we have outlined some benefits to working out with kettlebells, specifically for women:

- You can have a star quality body. Jennifer Lopez and Jennifer Aniston both workout with Kettlebells. These women have great bodies and you can too.

- Everyday tasks become easier. Physical Trainers call kettlebell training a "functional" workout. Functional means you are working your muscles the same way you do when you complete everyday tasks.

- You engage more muscles. When you swing the kettlebell in a pattern, you generate and regulate velocity. This action stimulates muscles in the legs, butt and abs during the entire workout.

- You will lose weight faster and decrease body fat. When you are activating multiple muscles at the same time you burn more calories. In a standard kettlebell training session a woman can burn about 20 calories per minute. Regularly working with kettlebells will help increase your metabolism and result in a decrease of body fat.

- You will discover that you are stronger than you imagined. It is recommended that women start with a 13-26 pound kettlebell. The combination of velocity and strength allow you to lift more weight than you are used to.

- It increases your strength without becoming bulky. Women usually do not want to start looking like body builders. Kettlebell workouts build up strength and increase lean muscle not muscle mass.

- Improving your posture. Posture is extremely important during kettlebell workouts, you back and abs should be straight at all times.

- Saves time. A great kettlebell workout can be done in just 15 minutes, every day.

Chapter 2. Tips for Choosing The Right Size Kettlebell

If you are just getting started in Kettlebell workouts, you want to purchase your own set of Kettlebells. Since Kettlebell's have become more popular there has been an increase in options for purchase. Here are some tips that you will want to consider when buying Kettlebells:

Tip #1 – Choose different sizes. Instead of just having one weight, buy different size weights. Some exercises are better with larger weights while others are better with smaller weights. Having 4 or 5 options will give you a good range for different workouts.

Tip #2 – Consider your Current Strength. Test a Kettlebell about five pounds less than the weight you are currently lifting. Try a few swings. It should be hard, but it should not hurt or feel like you will drop it easily.

Tip #3 – Lift before buying. You don't want to be struggling but it should not be effortless either.

Tip #4 – Recommended Weight. Women will often buy Kettlebells that are too light. Ballistic exercises recommend a weight of 18 to 26 pounds, and grinding exercises recommend 13 to 18 pounds. Important Note: If you are out of shape, selecting a lower weight is acceptable.

Chapter 3. Avoiding Dangerous Mistakes

No one wants to hurt themselves while working out. Kettlebells can be dangerous if not used properly; you or someone else could be injured. It is important to take certain things into consideration when participating in a Kettlebell Workout.

- Have Enough Space. If you are in a public gym, you need to be certain you have enough space. Injury can occur if another person gets to close.

- Do not Over Train. If you are training too much or too often you are at risk of muscle damage. Beginners should start with a lower intensity workout and then gradually increase.

- Keep your Spine Straight. Failing to keep a straight spine can cause serious injury to your back. If you can't keep straight then you need to decrease the weight of your kettlebell.

- Don't Grip to Tightly. This can cause sore hands and elbows; it can also raise your blood pressure.

- Be Sure to Keep an Athletic Stance. Overextending can put your back, knees, and hips at risk of injury.

- Don't Get Too Fancy. The basics really do work the best.

- Wear the Right Shoes. Kettlebell workouts are not meant for running shoes. You should wear flat soled shoes or bare feet. Running shoes could contribute to knee injuries.

Chapter 4. Getting Started with Kettlebells

Most large gyms do not offer kettlebells but smaller gyms and trainers usually have classes available. If you want to get started with kettlebells the best thing to do is locate a trainer who is kettlebell certified. You can learn the basics from DVDs or videos on the internet, but it is much healthier and safer to get one on one training to start off.

One on one training is recommended for those just starting with kettlebells because it takes a lot of body awareness and coordination to perform these exercises. With just one exercise you are working out a combination of muscles and joints, all at the same time. A trainer can teach you how to move properly with a kettlebell. As you noticed from our previous section there are a number of dangers that can occur from kettlebell workouts, so it is especially important you are trained right. It is a workout that takes time and plenty of practice to perfect. If these exercises are done incorrectly, there is risk for serious injury. Improperly done exercises can cause injury to your joints, back, neck or spine. It is important that you are making an effort to be safe.

There are a many different combinations and styles for holding your kettlebell. The following are a number of different Kettlebell and Hand Combinations:

Kettlebell Hand Combinations

1 Kettlebell – Held by 2 Hands

1 Kettlebell – Held by 1 Hand

2 Kettlebells – 1 Hand, holds both Kettlebells

2 Kettlebells – 2 Hands, each holds a Kettlebell

4 Kettlebells – 2 Hands, each holds 2 Kettlebells

Kettlebell Grips

Regular – The handle is held in the palm, kettlebell is on the outside of the arm.

Reverse – The handles is held in the palm, kettlebell is on the inside of the arm.

Horn – Bell is bottom down or up, hands are around the horns.

Horn Squeeze – Similar to above, but palms are squeezed together.

Two Hand Hold – Handle is held with both hands.

Horn (Taffy) Pull – Holding the horns with both hands, as if pulling apart.

Bottom Up – Handle is on the Bottom.

Two Hand, Bottom Up – Two hands, hold one bottom up kettlebell.

Waiter – When the kettlebell rests on an open palm, like a waiter holding a tray.

Farmers Hold – Wrists bent or straight with kettlebell on either side.

Foot in Handle – Your foot is in the handle.

How Long Should the Workout Last?

If you are engaging in resistance training you should only complete a 30 minute kettlebell workout. After 30 minutes you will lose your energy rapidly and your workout will become ineffective. If you have energy to carry on longer, then your workout wasn't hard enough to start. At 30 minutes your body will be operating on low energy, if you keep working out your stress level will rise.

If you are looking to burn calories and fat, with a cardio kettlebell workout you can train longer than 30 minutes. A steady cardio routine can last for about an hour without any negative effects. During this hour your workout should be slow and steady, high intensity training will result in fatigue and loss of muscle.

A thirty minute workout is a basic principal for most weight training. However your energy level can be affected by how much you eat before a workout, how long ago you ate, and what was eaten. It is important to use your time productively, push yourself and you are sure to see results.

How Often Should You Exercise with Kettlebells?

There is no one answer to this question. In fact it depends on; how long you have been training, what other training have you been doing, your goals, and etc.

If a kettlebell workout is the only regular workout you are doing than three times per week is suggested. For example; you could train one day, rest two, then train again and so on. It could look like this:

- Monday: Workout

- Tuesday: Rest

- Wednesday: Rest

- Thursday: Workout

- Friday: Rest

- Saturday: Rest

- Sunday: Workout

- Monday: Rest

This could continue on and on each week.

If you get to the point where you think you are ready for more, you can choose to rest only one day, and increase your workouts to four days a week. You will want to be sure to split up your routine so that you aren't working the same muscles each time. To split your workout routine effectively you can divide your body into sections. A good workout routine divides your body into three and offers a Push/Pull/Leg Split Exercise.

- Push Exercise – Any exercise with a push motion. Examples would be; chest, shoulder and triceps exercises like; bench pressing, overhead presses and triceps extensions.

- Pull Exercise – Any exercise with a pull motion. Your back and biceps muscles are worked during these exercises. Common exercises include; deadlift, rows, biceps curls.

- Legs – These are lower body movements to work your leg muscles. Exercises include; squats, lunges, pistols, leg deadlifts and calf raises.

Splitting your routine and breaking up your workout will allow your muscles time to repair and grow. If you still need or want to exercise in between time, do a completely different type of workout and allow your muscles to rest from the kettlebells. Maybe you think we forgot about your abs. Your abs will be worked out consistently in each workout because of the format for kettlebell training. So there is no need to split into an abs specific routine. It is important to remember that your muscles need rest in order to grow.

Chapter 5. Keys to Successful Kettlebell Workouts

It is important to make sure your program works, you want to formulate an effective workout plan. When planning a workout you should follow some guidelines in order to achieve the best possible results. If you are not seeing progress than you did not plan correctly.

1. Strength before Cardio. Most often when you exercise you complete conditioning first; you run, bike or use the elliptical. By the time you are finished you have already lost strength and energy, maybe your legs are even weak. Strength exercises should be completed first, it will help you improve physically.

2. Practice. You need to do multiple reps and do them well. Kettlebell moves can be confusing, practice and continue to improve your form and lifts.

3. Know when you're Not Ready. If you cannot properly perform a lift at a certain weight, then you need to move to the weight below. The more practice you have the better you will become. Be patient and enjoy the journey. Taking on more than you are ready for will only lead to injury.

4. Don't Attempt to Much. More than likely you are not an elite athlete or body builder, so don't attempt to train like one. Kettlebell training is a whole body exercise so there is no need to go overboard and do every workout available. If you are going to pick multiple exercises, pick ones that complement each other.

5. Pace Yourself. The whole reason you are training is to build up your body for the long haul, if you expend all your energy right away every time you will not be able to continue for long. You shouldn't go to easy on yourself either, find the right balance.

A good productive workout requires hard work and patience. If you want to see results you have to put in the time and be willing to wait for results. Plan your workout and set goals so that you have the best opportunity for success.

Kettlebell Training Styles

There are two main styles of Kettlebell training. Hard Style or RKC, this style uses explosive power in the technique. Tension is created, in order to exert more strength. Soft Style or AKC is more relaxed to complete more repetitions. There is less tension and more softness in the technique.

Chapter 6. Common Kettlebell Movements

Kettlebell workouts are great because they work the entire body with their off centered weight. Increasing the work of your muscles is key to burning calories. Kettlebell can help you achieve your fitness goals and get results. Here are some of the most common kettlebell movements:

- **Kettlebell Swing:** This move involves almost all of the muscles in your body, targeting the back, abs, hips, butt, legs and shoulders. In this move you stand with your feet slightly wider than hip width apart, knees slightly bent and back straight. Grab the kettlebell with two hands between your legs at knee height and swing in a controlled upwards motion, above your head, arms straight. Bring the kettlebell back down between your legs in a controlled manner. This swinging motion should last about 20 seconds each repetition.

- **Kettlebell Goblet Squat:** This movement works the leg and butt muscles. Hold your weight at your chest, your elbows should face down at the floor and your arms should be almost vertical. Slowly, lower into the squat position. Your elbows should touch your inner thighs. Pause after the squat is completed and then shoot upwards and activate your butt muscles. Do not move the kettlebell during this move, your legs are doing all the movements. Again, your back should be straight and do not bend forward.

- **Standing Pull Up:** With this movement you will stand with your feet apart. Start with your weight, being held at the bottom of your straight arms. Pull up your elbows and keep your arms tight. You should feel the work out in your shoulders.

- **Single Arm Rows:** For this movement you should be kneeling on a bench, one foot to the floor. Your back should be straight and your shoulders should be even; brace your core. With your hand, pick the kettlebell off the floor and row upwards. Your elbow should point at the ceiling, and then lower the weight back to the starting point.

- **Triceps Extension:** This kettlebell movement will work your abs and triceps. Place one foot in front of another. Keep your shoulders back and back straight. Pick up the kettlebell with both hands, lift it over your head, make your elbows tight and slowly lower the weight behind your head, then bring it back up. Keep control over the weight and don't let it fall back quickly.

- One Arm Press: For this movement you will need to be in the plank position, with each hand on a kettlebell. Keep your back straight, butt tight and pull on kettlebell towards your body like a row. When you get to the top, squeeze and return to start, and switch sides.

- Windmill: Similar to the shoulder press but with two additional movements. Complete the press movement and then angle your feet, keeping your arms straight, lock your elbow. The arm with the weight goes to the top and the other arm will go to the ground, creating a windmill shape. The slower you being the better. Keep your spine straight and look straight ahead. Exhale when you come back and move back into the shoulder press and continue with another rep.

- Bent over Row: Use two kettlebells for this exercise; place them between your feet. Slightly bend your knees and push your butt out, as if you were sitting on a chair. Pick up both weights and bring them to your stomach. Bring the bells back down and repeat. Keep control.

- **Figure 8:** This move targets the arm, back and abdominal muscles. Your legs should be slightly wider than hip-width apart, and lower to a quarter squat. Hold the kettlebell with your left hand and swing it around the left leg and between the legs, pass to the right hand and swing it around the right leg. Continue this motion for your intended rep, switch directions about half way through the rep. Similar to the Figure-8 basketball drill.

- **Kettlebell Lunge Press:** These lunges will work on your shoulders, back, arm, butt, ab, and leg muscles. With this movement you should stand straight, place the kettlebell at your chest with both hands, and keep arms bent and your palms facing each other. Do a stationary lunge with one leg and bring the kettlebell above the head. Move back into the standing position and bring the kettlebell back to your chest. Be sure to keep your movements controlled.

- **Deadlift:** This advanced move works your legs, butt, arms, back and abdominals. The kettlebell should be on the floor between your feet. Squat and hold the

26

kettlebell with two hands. Keep your back straight. Rise up, with your arms extended. Your core should be engaged, butt should be tight and back should be straight. This move should be controlled. Slowly squat back down and bring the weight back down to the starting position and repeat.

- **Kettlebell Half Get-Up:** Work your abdominal muscles, arms and back with this move. Lie on your back with your legs out. With the kettlebell lift your right arm straight up. Bend the left knee and rise, your left arm will keep your body propped. If your abs are burning, you are doing it right. Return to the start position and switch sides.

- **Push Ups:** This is as simple as it sounds. Do a push up while holding onto your kettlebells. Holding onto the kettlebells is a lot harder than having your hands flat on the floor.

- **Orbit:** Hold your kettlebell by the handle and get into bottoms up position. Orbit your head in a smooth motion with the kettlebell. If one elbow is up the other is down.

- Sling Short or Around the Body Pass: This movement is done in the standing position. Keeping your back straight and shoulders back swing the kettlebell around your body, change hands in the front and back of your body. You want your elbows to be as straight as possible.

Chapter 7. Kettlebell Workouts

Basic Kettlebell Workout

This workout starts with just five basic movements. It is a great way to get started and learn to practice the movements. Once you have conquered this routine, move on to something more difficult. A 5 or 10 pound kettlebell is recommended for beginners. This circuit is just five moves, complete 10 reps on each move. The circuit should be completed three times.

As you become stronger you can increase weights or repetitions but you want to start low and work your way up. It is important to focus on your form first. When you can do 20 reps of each of these moves correctly, then you should increase your weight. Be sure to pace yourself, and listen to your body.

Move #1 – Swing

Move #2 – Figure 8

Move #3 – Windmill

Move #4 – Halo

Move #5 – Orbit

The Killer Kettlebell Workout

This workout is great for women that love kettlebells. These simple pieces of equipment can help sculpt your entire body. This workout will work your shoulders, back, butt, abs and arms. With this routine you will engage in eight back to back kettlebell movements. Once circuits are complete rest for one or two minutes and then repeat for two or three circuits. A 10 to 15 pound kettlebell should be sufficient for most women. Follow this routine 2 to 3 days per week.

1. Around the Body Pass (At your Waist) – 10 Reps
2. Bent Row – 10 to 12 Reps
3. Dead Lift – 10 to 12 Reps
4. Figure 8 (Between your Legs) – 10 Reps
5. Half Get Ups – 5 Reps
6. Swing – 15 to 20 Reps
7. Front Squats – 10 to 15 Reps
8. Windmill – 5 to 10 Reps

Bell Curves: A 20 Minute Interval Kettlebell Workout

This workout is great for women who don't have a lot of time to accomplish cardio and strength training workout. With this workout you will get the best of both worlds. You will need a 5 to 15 pound kettlebell depending upon your experience. Burn 240 calories with this 20 minute workout.

Step 1 – Jog in place for 1 minute, then do Jumping Jacks for 1 minute. Total Time = 2 minutes

Step 2 – Kettlebell Swing, do 6 to 7 reps of 10. Total Time = 2 Minutes.

Step 3 – Knee Highs. Total Time = 2 Minutes.

Step 4 – Stationary Lunges with Kettlebell, alternating legs. Total Time = 2 Minutes.

Step 5 – Squat Jump with Kettlebell. Total Time = 1 Minute.

Step 6 – Kettlebell Figure 8. Total Time = 1 Minute.

Step 7 – Repeat Steps 2 thru 6. Total Time = 8 Minutes.

Step 8 – March in Place while doing Arm Circles. Alternate forward and backward motion. Total Time = 2 Minutes.

Advanced Workout for Women

This workout is not for beginners. It is a full body workout for both strength and conditioning. These three sets of exercises will challenge your whole body. No resting between exercises but you can rest for 30 to 60 seconds between circuits.

Circuit A1 – Thrusters: 3 sets of 60 seconds.

Circuit A2 – Figure 8: 3 sets of 60 seconds.

Circuit A3 – Overhead Sit Up: 3 sets of 60 seconds.

Circuit B1 – Gorilla Leap: 3 sets of 60 seconds.

Circuit B2 – High Pull (Alternating): 3 sets of 60 seconds.

Circuit B3 – Half TGU: 3 sets of 60 seconds.

Circuit C1 – Push Up: 3 sets of 60 seconds.

Circuit C2 – Swing (Alternating): 3 sets of 60 seconds.

Circuit C3 – Gladiator Hold: 3 sets of 30 seconds each side.

Kettlebell Body Challenge Workout for Women

This is an intense kettlebell workout for those who have been progressing in their skills. Follow this circuit routine and repeat four to five times. This routine can be done 3 to 4 times per week, with a weight that is suitable for your skill level.

- 10 Push Ups

- 10 Swings

- 10 Squats (Sumo Style)

- 45 Second Rest

- 15 Push Ups

- 15 Swings

- 15 Squats (Sumo Style)

- 45 Second Rest

- 20 Push Ups

- 20 Swings

- 20 Squats (Sumo Style)

- 45 Second Rest and Repeat

This workout is progressive; it increases in interval sets helping with strength training. If the challenge is too much decrease the number of circuits or the amount of weight you are using.

Conclusion

At first glance the kettlebell doesn't look like anything special. This book clearly shows the power and capabilities of this small cast-iron piece of exercise equipment. With just this one piece of equipment you can get a complete and total body workout, in just thirty minutes. You can work your back, arms, legs, butt and abdominal muscles with just this one piece of equipment.

Be sure to consult a certified kettlebell trainer before attempting these exercises on your own. Although it may be tempting to try the many number of videos available online, this small weight can be dangerous if not used properly. Get proper training for your safety and the safety of others. Take your time, be safe and you will feel your body change. Work hard, be diligent and you will see the results you are looking for.

Thank You Page

I want to personally thank you for reading my book. I hope you found information in this book useful and I would be very grateful if you could leave your honest review about this book. I certainly want to thank you in advance for doing this.